Butterfly Gone Rogue

Butterfly Gone Rogue

Mansi Sagar

Life Rattle Press Toronto, Canada

Butterfly Gone Rogue

Life Rattle Press, Toronto, Canada
Stories copyright © 2020 by Mansi Sagar

Library and Archives Canada Cataloguing in Publication

Butterfly Gone Rogue / Mansi Sagar. -- First Canadian edition.
Life Rattle New Publishers Series, ISSN 978-1-897161-84-5
Short Stories
ISBN 978-1-989861-01-1

Cover Design by Celine Polidario
Copy Edit by Nick West
Typeset by Mansi Sagar

To Pappa and Mummy

Contents

Last Exam..1

Tests..5

The Only Choice...11

Indeterminate...17

Surgery...25

Waking Up...31

The Hospital Stay...37

Back Home...45

Surprise..53

Two Point Six Millimeters.....................................57

The Butterfly Necklace..61

Cancer is Not a Dirty Word....................................69

Last Exam

Hey, we are going for a walk, Pappa says as he strokes his salt and pepper beard. "When is your exam?"

"The day after," I answer.

Pappa wears a half-sleeved, pastel-colored shirt with long, dark pants. He sports an oversized watch on his left wrist, a silver bracelet on his right wrist, and a white gold ring on his left index finger. He smells of his favorite Armani cologne.

"Okay, do you want take-out? We will be back in an hour or so," Pappa asks.

"Naah, I'm okay," I reply.

Pappa and Mummy put on their shoes and head out the door. Since Pappa is semi-retired and Mummy is a housewife, they go for walks around the neighborhood to kill time and get their daily cardio.

The sunlight stings my eyes through the large floor-to-ceiling windows. My laptop lies on a pile of notes on the wooden dining table. CP24 anchors mumble in the background. It's noon, and I start studying for my Anthropology exam. I push in my earbuds and stare at my laptop screen.

I stroke the front of my neck with my right hand while I read over the notes. I feel an oval-shaped bump sticking out.

Over the next few hours, I feel it grow. I find the back of my neck stiff.

I had hypothyroidism, a thyroid disease, when I was in high school. I stroke the lump and Google "thyroid in body" and head over to the images.

I see real-life pictures and anatomy diagrams. I learn that my thyroid gland—also known as a butterfly gland because of its striking resemblance to the winged creature—wraps around my trachea.

I send a picture to the "Sagar Sisters" group chat.

"I have this sticking out," I say and wait for my older sisters, Kiran Didi and Tanvi Didi, to reply. They don't respond quickly. Kiran Didi lives in the U.K. with her husband and kids and Tanvi Didi lives in Bahrain with hers.

Mummy and Pappa return from their walk and I tell them about my discovery. Mummy scans the lump first and asks Pappa to take a closer look. They stare at my neck intently as if they have X-ray vision.

"You should go see Dr. Kothari about this," Pappa replies.

"I will, I need to study for my exam," I say.

"It will keep bugging you. Book an appointment right now," Pappa replies.

Pappa always wants things done now. He does not believe in "tomorrow" or "in an hour" or "in a minute." If Pappa asks me to do something, he expects me to do it right away.

The next day, I feel discomfort, and the lump feels hard.

I Google "lump on thyroid" and get results of nodules and

thyroid cancer. The WebMD website reassures me that I have 90% chance of it being benign. I exhale. I click back over to my notes.

I barge into Pappa and Mummy's bedroom and sit on their king-size bed. I feel that my voice cracks. Hoarseness is a sign of thyroid cancer, based on WebMD. Pappa is hunched over at his desktop computer.

"Do you think I sound different?" I ask Pappa.

"No, why?" He glances at me.

"I'm just asking." I stroke the back of the left side of my neck as my muscles cramp.

"Take an Advil and book an appointment with Dr. Kothari," he says.

I gulp down an Advil. I call up Dr. Kothari and book an appointment.

It's the day of my exam. I scan over my notes.

"Do you want me to drop you off at UTM for your exam?" Pappa asks as he strokes his oversized belly after lunch. I notice the tiny daal stain on his white shirt and then at his bald head.

When he was younger, he loved combing his hair, that's what Mummy told me. I have never seen him with a full head of hair. Now, he just strokes his bald head with Mummy's comb.

He inhales his vape. The smell of spices, herbs, and cooked vegetables in the apartment overpowers the Armani cologne he wears. Harsh, minty tobacco smoke—with a hint of fennel—escapes his mouth as he exhales. I gather my pile of notes and cradle my laptop.

"Yes, please, we can leave in two hours," I respond. "I feel better, but I don't think I can bus it."

"It might be because of the Advil. I'll be napping then. You'll have to bus," Pappa sounds tired.

Pappa suffers from type two diabetes and cataracts. In his sixties, his body struggles. He's on medications which make him drowsy and fatigued. He needs to take his naps to re-charge and does not like skipping them. Siestas were a part of his lifestyle when we lived in Bahrain because of the work culture there. Now it's become a necessity.

Pappa asks if I need a ride to school or if I need to be picked up once in a while. I think he misses being my Pappa. Pappa started to offer rides after he became semi-retired, since he was busy running his business while I was growing up. If Pappa and I fight, he makes up for it through small gestures like giving me rides or getting my favourite take-outs.

"Pappa, please?" I beg. I feel tired.

"Okay fine," Pappa agrees.

I head over to my room, plop on my bed and continue cramming.

Tests

On a windy April morning, I enter a cubicle-like room and take a seat on a stiff, metal chair with sparse padding. The room contains an examination table, informational posters plastered to the light blue walls, and a small sink with a floral hand-wash.

I stare at the child-painted Mona Lisa imitation framed on the wall.

I squint at the computer screen and notice my last name written in tiny letters.

Dr. Kothari struts in and collapses into her swiveling chair. She beams, and her off-white teeth peek out.

"So, what brings you in today?" She asks.

"I have this lump, wanted to get it checked," I reply, as I stroke my neck.

She adjusts her glasses on the bridge of her nose, brings her chair closer, and touches the lump.

"Hmm, do you have any symptoms such as difficulty breathing or muscular pain?" She applies gentle pressure.

"Muscular pain yes, it expands and contracts and my shoulders and neck ache," I reply.

"Okay, it's probably a cyst," she says.

I roll my eyes. I don't think a lump this hard is a cyst.

She turns back to her computer and pulls up my file.

"A large nodule on the left side of her neck, possibly a cyst." She mumbles as she types.

"We will get an ultrasound done and also a fine needle aspiration...a biopsy. Let me also refer you to a head and neck surgeon," she says as she looks into my eyes and struts out.

I follow her. The assistant hands me printed requisition forms.

I head home.

The next day, I arrive for my ultrasound. I follow a practitioner who instructs me to lie on the examination table and extend my neck.

I stretch my neck back and examine where the ceiling intersects with the wall. The practitioner covers my top with paper towels, spreads cool gooey jelly on my neck, and places the ultrasound probe on my nodule. She types and clicks the mouse as she stares at the screen. I peek at the monitor. I see grayscale objects with red and blue blots.

"Alright, it's probably a benign nodule on your thyroid." The practitioner says. "Your family doctor will give you further information...you're all done, use paper towels to clean up your neck,"

I wipe the water-based goo from my neck and stride out.

. . .

A week later, I wait in the same cubicle-like room at Dr. Kothari's office.

I wish Pappa or Mummy had come along, even if they sat outside in the waiting room.

I fidget with my long nails.

Dr. Kothari struts in and hops on her seat.

"Okay let's see your ultrasound results," she says.

"It's a big nodule and it is part of your thyroid. It's about five centimeters big." She says. "I think a biopsy should let us know for sure, we will get you a date but most likely it's benign." She squints at the screen.

I exhale. I wish she could tell me the exact diagnosis.

I march out and drive home.

When I get home, I tell Pappa the news. He nods.

"When did she say you will get the biopsy date?" Pappa asks.

"Probably in a few months. Why does it take so long for the goddamn healthcare? Urgh. I just want to know what this is." I whine. "I also forgot to pick up the blood work requisition."

"If it's an emergency, they do stuff quick. For now, they think it's benign," Pappa replies.

"Hmm… can you come with me to my biopsy appointment? I won't be able to drive back afterwards. Based on my research, it's not recommended," I say to Pappa.

"Probably, but that depends on my nap time. How do you know that you won't be able to drive back afterwards?" Pappa says.

"I read stuff online. They poke you with a long needle while they scan your neck with an ultrasound probe. I have to stay still. No sound. No movement…" I say.

"Okay, I will come with you. You will be fine," Pappa promises. "Just give me the address, as soon as you get it. Call Dr. Kothari and ask for the requisition. Pick it up tomorrow."

"I don't want to go tomorrow," I say.

"Call her up and ask," Pappa insists. "We can get your blood work done after we get groceries."

. . .

On a sunny June afternoon, two months after my first appointment, Mummy and I get dropped off at the main entrance of the Medical Building near Credit Valley Hospital.

"I told you we should've left earlier. It's just five minutes to my appointment," I say as I get out of the car.

Pappa mouths a response and drives off to the parking lot.

Pappa does not mind if he walks in five minutes late to an appointment.

"Doctors always run late," he says. He is right. But I prefer to be punctual.

Mummy takes a seat in the crowded waiting area while I wait in line. The smell of sweat and hand sanitizer fill the room. Mummy gets busy with her phone.

Pappa walks in and grabs a seat. He stares at his oversized phone and adjusts his glasses. He glances at me and back at the phone. He gulps and scrolls. I'm happy I have Mummy and Pappa here.

"Yo, is the place at the main hospital?" Nudrat texts on WhatsApp.

"It's at the small building next to it. It's downstairs. Call me when you get here." I text back.

Nudrat is a friend from UTM. She wants to be present at my biopsy appointment. She understands it is a serious procedure. She had a relative die due to a biopsy complication.

Once I finish registering, I spot an empty seat opposite

Mummy and take it.

"Do you have anything to eat?" Pappa asks Mummy.

Mummy searches her bag.

Pappa needs to eat something every few hours. His sugar levels fluctuate if he does not rest or eat, which makes him groggy.

Nudrat's caller ID lights up my phone. I walk out and accept the call.

"Yo, I'm coming in two minutes, waiting for the elevator," Nudrat says.

I hang up. I take a deep breath and wait for her by the door.

Five minutes later, Nudrat comes in with a bouquet of sunflowers and hugs me.

A few minutes later, I go in for my biopsy.

The Only Choice

Two months after my biopsy, we arrive at the head and neck surgeon Dr. Dobrowski's clinic. August sunshine brightens the waiting area. Kids play with colorful plastic toys in the middle of the waiting room. Chairs with watchful parents line the play area.

Pappa and I wait for my appointment.

A little girl walks out of Dr. Dobrowski's office. She wails and stuffs a tissue up her nose. The kids at the play area get distracted and stare at her.

I text my friend, Mihir. We recently started talking after a few years. We had drifted apart. He lives in India.

"Mansi Sagar," Dr, Dobrowski yells.

I jump up from my seat and walk towards her.

"Hey," Dr. Dobrowski says as she ushers me into her office.

I hop on an elevated chair in the middle of the room. Its brown leather reminds me of electrocution chairs like the ones you see in creepy TV shows. Pappa sits opposite me and Dr. Dobrowski stands beside me. Pappa taps his foot and clasps his hands together.

"So, what brought you in today?" Dr. Dobrowski asks.

"I got referred because I have this," I stroke the lump.

She reaches for my neck.

"It's hard and very big…" She glances at her notes. "Good news is that the biopsy came back benign." She pokes my nodule.

I glance over at Pappa as he scans the pile of folders stacked in a corner. Pappa glances at me, then at Dr. Dobrowski and exhales.

"Because it is a big nodule, the only way to get it out is surgery," Dr. Dobrowski says.

"Is that the only option? What about laser?" Pappa stares at Dr. Dobrowski. His eyebrows lift, and his nostrils flare. He scratches his forehead and glances at me.

"No. That's the only option…I will refer you to a fellow surgeon. I need to check your voice box and look for any obstructions." She takes out a thin, black one-foot long pipe with a small built-in camera torch at one end and a screen at the other.

I stare into Pappa's eyes. He stares back and exhales. He blinks and smiles. I try to smile and clench my fists.

"Okay Mansi, I am going to put this in through your nose. Stay still, it will make you feel teary-eyed and funny when it comes out."

The pipe shimmies up my nostril and down my trachea like a snake. My mouth opens up.

Pappa tries to peek at the screen. He looks at the pipe and I glance at the bridge of my nose. Sweat droplets trickle down my back.

She stares at the screen and removes the pipe. As it comes out of my nose, my eyes well and I sneeze.

"Okay, it looks clear." She hands me a tissue. "Have a great day." She leads us out and calls her next patient in.

"I feel funny," I say. "Were you not scared when she put the pipe inside me?"

"Nope, when you were in an incubator, you were fed through a tube inserted in your nose at every feeding," Pappa replies, remembering my premature birth at thirty-one weeks.

Mummy told me Pappa used to drive three to four times a day to visit me at the neo-natal clinic. Pappa used to juggle his three kids, his business and visiting Mummy and I at the hospital. Mummy told me he used to visit me more than her. I think Pappa now gets tired of visiting the doctors.

We stare at the lit-up elevator button.

"Can you drive?" I ask.

Pappa glances over at me. "Yes," he sighs. "Call Mummy and tell her."

. . .

Two months later, chilly October winds hit us as we enter the medical building at Credit Valley Hospital, two days after my twentieth birthday. We enter Dr. Wazir's office. He's a general surgeon. Middle-aged people stare at their phones in the waiting room. The chairs surround a coffee table cluttered with crumpled magazines and informational pamphlets.

"Okay, I'm going in. I will let you know what happens," I message Mihir as I get called in.

"Cool, it will all be fine, don't worry," Mihir replies.

I walk towards the door. Pappa follows. Mummy waits in the waiting area and scrolls through the messages on her phone.

I knock. Dr. Wazir organizes papers on his desk and smiles

at us. His overgrown beard catches my attention.

"Hello, take a seat," Dr. Wazir says.

Pappa and I sit on the two chairs opposite Dr. Wazir.

"Your nodule looks big. Is it okay if I take a look?" Dr. Wazir asks.

I nod and remove my wool scarf and tie my hair up.

Dr. Wazir stands behind me. He squishes my neck.

"So where do you study?" He asks.

"UTM," I sound breathless.

He finishes with my neck and jumps onto his chair.

"Because it's big, we will either have to do a lobectomy, to remove the left lobe, or a total thyroidectomy, to remove the whole gland." Dr. Wazir says. "Regarding complications, there's a minute chance you may lose your voice, but it is not common. Also, if your parathyroid glands get damaged, you may experience low calcium levels."

Pappa and I nod.

"Because of your age and the size of it, there's a higher chance that it could be cancer. I want to perform another biopsy." Dr. Wazir says.

Pappa and I stare into his insistent eyes and look back at each other.

"If you could follow me to the next room," Dr. Wazir stretches his hand at the door and smiles as we follow him out.

I remove my jacket and hand it over to Pappa. I lie straight on the examining table and Pappa plops onto a stiff chair. The smell of hand sanitizer overpowers the room.

Dr. Wazir prepares his needle at the corner work-station.

"Stay still." He stands behind me and leans forward. "Just a slight pinch."

I nod.

He pokes me. The needle pushes into my nodule. He is assertive as he probes with the needle in all directions. His scrubs graze my forehead.

He paces back to his work station and inserts the contents into a sterile container. He returns and waves the sterile container above my face. I glance at the tiny white tissues floating in clear liquid.

He places a Band-Aid on my nodule.

"Wait for ten minutes here and then Kim, my assistant, will give you more information. I'll see you in two weeks." He exits the room.

Pappa and I wait. My feet dangle. I face Pappa. He smiles.

"How did it feel?" He asks.

"Worse than the first biopsy...were you not grossed out?" I ask.

"It was cool," Pappa says. "He has good hands."

"Yeah." My throat scratches.

"What do you want to eat later on?" Pappa asks.

"Can you make pasta your way?" I ask.

"Sure," Pappa replies.

Pappa loves to cook. Most days, he helps Mummy in the kitchen.

"Can you help me with my jacket?" I get down from the

examining table.

Pappa holds my jacket and helps me put my hands through.

We exit the room, notify Kim and book our next appointment.

"What happened?" Mummy asks.

"Dr. Wazir performed a biopsy," I complain.

Mummy rubs my hand and gives me a quick hug.

We head out.

"I hope it comes out benign," I say, strolling beside Pappa.

"It will. The last one was benign." He swings his arms as he marches. "Call up Kiran and Tanvi right now, let's tell them."

Indeterminate

It is late October and cold rain droplets plummet onto the ground as grey clouds obstruct the sun.

Dr. Vernier, my endocrinologist, studies the computer screen as he hunts for my biopsy file. I look at the empty seat beside me and at him. He strokes his chin. He scans the biopsy report that I am supposed to find out about through Dr. Wazir.

"Indeterminate and inconclusive." Dr. Vernier continues. "With a higher chance of it being cancer."

I exit Dr. Vernier's office. Pappa and Mummy follow. The rain dampens the frizzy fish-braid that Mummy tied for me.

"Pappa, can you drive please?" I mumble.

"Sure," Pappa replies.

In 2017, Dr. Vernier told me that I may have trouble having babies and may develop further health issues due to polycystic ovary syndrome. I was eighteen. After my visit, I opened up to Mummy and Pappa.

"It's alright, you can always adopt, everything will be fine" Pappa said as he drove home.

"It will be okay, Mansi," Mummy said and stared out the window.

I think about Dr. Vernier's words. I open the car door and

jump in. The smells of wet mud and damp air collide with the minty car freshener.

Pappa gets into the driver's seat and Mummy eases herself onto the front passenger seat. They spin to face me.

"So, what did Dr. Vernier say?" Pappa asks.

"The result came out indeterminate...there is a higher chance of it being cancerous," I attempt to speak.

Pappa's eyes bulge and he freezes.

"But, how?" He gulps "Are you sure? I should've come inside with you," he replies.

Tears overflow, and I wail.

"Don't cry" Pappa pats my shoulder and says in a faint voice. "We will do more tests, okay?" He clears his throat.

Mummy hands me a box of tissues.

"Mansi, everything will be fine." Mummy says.

I grab a tissue, blow my nose, and wipe my tears with my frozen fingers.

"Call Tanvi and Kiran," Pappa says to Mummy in Gujarati.

Mummy WhatsApp calls Kiran Didi. Pappa starts the engine and drives. The windshield wipers toss the water off the front window.

"Hi, what are you guys up to?" Kiran Didi says.

"Yeah, talk to Mansi," Mummy says as she hands the phone over.

"I can't do it," I hand the phone back to Mummy. I sniffle and gulp.

"I will pass it on to Pappa," Mummy faces the phone towards Pappa.

I unlock my phone and go to Mihir's message. I inform him about the result.

Pappa projects his voice. "Yes, Kiran, so Mansi's second biopsy came out indeterminate."

"What does that mean?" Kiran Didi asks.

"Not sure. It's not benign." Pappa answers.

"It will be okay," Mummy interrupts.

Tears flow down my cheeks, snot drips from my nose, and I dab it with a tissue. My watery eyes fog my glasses and obstruct my vision.

"Hmm...are you okay?" Kiran Didi asks.

"We have to be strong." Pappa replies.

"Mansi is strong," Mummy says in Gujarati.

"Where's Mansi?" Kiran Didi asks.

I stare unfocused, at the seat pocket in front of me.

Mummy hands me the phone and my eyes meet Kiran Didi's eyes on the screen. Tears escape. I gasp for air.

"Mansi, calm down...it's gonna be okay." She says. "Let's add Tanvi."

The call splits into three screens.

"Yeah, what's up people?" Tanvi Didi comes on screen and says.

I purse my lips.

"Mansi, what happened?" Tanvi Didi says.

"Her second biopsy came out indeterminate. It's neither benign nor cancerous," Kiran Didi says.

"Mansi, it will be okay," Tanvi Didi's smile faints.

"Let's take crazy pictures," Kiran Didi proposes.

Tanvi Didi stretches the tip of her nose upwards. She sticks her tongue out. Kiran Didi follows. She bulges her eyes out and crosses them. I wipe my tears and follow. I extend the tip of my nose upwards. I smile and my teeth peek.

Mummy glances back and smiles. Pappa glances at me from the rear-view mirror and chuckles.

· · ·

A week later, November arrives. Whistling wind blows fallen leaves. My gaze shifts from the ceiling-to-floor windows to the grey wooden floor beneath my bare feet. My pyjama bottoms almost touch the floor. A pile of lobectomy surgery documents lies on the dining table. I stare at the "Your Medical Journey" booklet.

I want the surgery to take place over the summer.

"You want to wait six months for cancer?" Dr. Wazir questioned.

"How long I can wait?" I asked.

"Two months maximum," Dr. Wazir replied.

After discussing with Dr. Wazir, Pappa and I decide on lobectomy in early January.

Pappa settles on his reclining chair and inhales his vape. He passes the vape to Mummy and she puffs as they watch a documentary on tigers.

"Pappa, is lobectomy the right choice of surgery?" I ask.

"Well...there is no right choice here. It would be worse if we made no choice, just like Dr. Wazir said," Pappa replies.

"Pappa, what if it's cancer? Then I will have to undergo surgery again for total removal. If I opt for that initially and it turns out benign, then I will be on lifelong medication in vain," I say.

"Mansi, everything will turn out fine," Mummy replies.

The last time Mummy heard the word "cancer", it was her grandma. She was diagnosed with blood cancer. Mummy was a kid. She told me how she fetched a bucket of soil for her grandma as blood gushed out of her nose often. Then she'd bury the bloody soil.

"Mansi, even if you lose the entire gland, you will be able to lead a normal life. Many people rely on lifelong thyroid medication. How about we text Kiran, Tanvi and Raju and get their opinions? Kiran has a friend who's a doctor." Pappa replies.

Raju Bhai, my cousin is a doctor himself and we ask for his advice on medical issues all the time.

"You ask them, I don't want to," I say.

Pappa stomps to the fridge and grabs a can of ginger ale and leftover curry. He opens the can and slurps. He microwaves the curry. I don't like the aroma.

"Okay, let's see what they say. For now, lobectomy is the right choice. You have chosen something, it's better than not doing anything." Pappa says.

The microwave beeps. Pappa grabs his can and leftover curry and sits on his reclining chair .

"Mansi's second biopsy result came indeterminate. What is the better option? Total thyroidectomy or lobectomy?" Pappa sends an audio message to Raju Bhai.

Pappa inhales his vape and exhales. He gobbles the curry. He zones out as he watches a tiger chase a helpless lone zebra.

. . .

It is the beginning of December. Pappa asks me to sit on the couch.

"So, are you happy with the decision of going for a lobectomy?" Pappa asks.

"I'm not sure," I answer.

"Why not?" He asks.

"Because Pappa, what if it's the wrong choice? I don't want to regret it." I lower my gaze.

"Let's look at the facts, Dr. Wazir said in his medical note you have a fifty percent or higher chance of it being cancer. Raju chose total thyroidectomy. Dr. Kothari said to trust your surgeon too," Pappa says.

"Alright, what do you think?" I ask him.

"Mansi, you have to trust your surgeon. What's stopping you?" He asks.

"I wish I knew my diagnosis." My eyebrows tense and I fold my arms.

"See, it's a spectrum. You're in the middle. I don't think there's any going back to benign," Pappa says.

"So, you think I should go for total thyroidectomy?" I ask him.

"Do you think it's convenient if you go through two surgeries within six months? Even you don't want that. Go with total thyroidectomy. Thyroid pills are very common," Pappa replies.

I breathe out and nod.

"Did you ask Kim, Dr. Wazir's assistant, how long you have until you change your mind on the type of surgery?" Pappa asks.

"Yeah, she said a month. So, before December 14th," I say.

My lobectomy is scheduled for January 14th, 2019.

"Alright, so call her up. I know I said any decision is good a month ago, but based on what I've heard from the doctors, now total thyroidectomy seems like the best decision," Pappa says.

I nod.

Two days later, I visit Dr. Wazir's office and change the surgery to a total thyroidectomy.

Surgery

On January the 14th at 5:30 am, we exit the basement garage. Pappa accelerates to go up the slope in the driveway onto the street. The sky is pitch black. The moon hides behind grey clouds. Pappa increases the volume of the song "High Hopes" by Panic! at the Disco. Mummy is zoned out and stares out the window.

I fold my arms and frown. I gaze out the window and ponder the next few hours. My lips quiver, I clench my teeth, and tears form.

"Have you printed out the form for UTM? We need to get it signed by your surgeon," Pappa asks.

"Yeah." I wipe a tear off my cheek.

I open my backpack, take out the form and scan it to double check.

I need to declare my absence from classes due to surgery. It says to get it signed by a surgeon, a nurse, or a doctor. It also mentions not to get it signed before or after the fact.

"It says that I won't be able to get it signed before or after the surgery, which means I won't be able to get it signed tomorrow," I say.

"That's not what it says," Pappa replies.

"Pappa, it literally says before or after the fact," I yell. I wish

I could run back home.

His eyebrows tense. He grips the steering wheel tight and turns right into the parking lot on the intersection of Eglinton and Confederation.

"No, it doesn't. Let me read it." Pappa's voice echoes.

"Can you two stop?" Mummy's voice deepens.

He glares into my eyes and snatches the paper from my hand. He turns on the interior light.

"You can't get it signed before your surgery. A few days after surgery is fine, but not too long after surgery." Pappa replies.

Pappa hands the form to Mummy.

I wipe my tears and stare out the window at the empty roads. I message Mihir about what happened, and he consoles me.

We reach Credit Valley Hospital at 6:00 am. We enter and wait at the surgery registration area. I glance at the closed Second Cup and crave muffins. A few minutes later, a receptionist wraps the hospital band around my wrist. We head for surgery prep at 7:00 am. I change into a gown and a robe. Pappa and I enter another cubicle-like room at 7:30 am, where they weigh me, and I gulp down two Tylenol's.

"Is that your mom?" The nurse asks as we stroll out.

Mummy glances at me and at the nurse. She holds my backpack.

"Yes," I reply.

"How about you give your mom a big hug, you are going to the surgery waiting area," the nurse replies.

Mummy's eyes well and tears escape. She holds my face and

gives me a quick peck on my cheek. I hug her tight and dig my face into her shoulder. I inhale the floral perfume that I love. Mummy sniffs and weeps on my shoulder. I cry. I hold Mummy and she holds my elbow.

"Good luck kiddo." She covers her mouth and sinks on her seat.

Pappa and I follow the nurse. She guides us to our seats while I sniffle.

Other patients wait for surgery. They converse and giggle with their loved ones. I hear mumbles between Dr. Wazir and his team as they discuss my surgery in an open space, office-like area. They flip through pages of documents.

"Why did she delay the surgery?" One person asks.

"I think it is cancer," another person adds.

"Yeah, I think so too," Dr. Wazir replies.

Pappa sits beside me.

The nurse hands me a tissue box and a warm blanket. Pappa adjusts the blanket on my knees.

"It's going to be okay." The nurse says. "Think happy thoughts. You know, there's a study which shows that if you think positive thoughts, you recover faster."

A mother walks in cradling her toddler. The toddler might be going in for surgery.

I wipe my tears. Pappa lets out a faint smile.

Pappa hands me another tissue. I blow my nose and hand it back to Pappa.

"You will be fine. Why did you start crying?" Pappa asks.

"Because Mummy did!" I complain.

"You're such a strong girl, come on, let's take a picture." Pappa extends his arm and I lean into his shoulder. He sends it to the WhatsApp Family group chat. It's 7:45 am.

Mummy has saved a carry-on bag filled with the family's old photos. Most of them are pictures of me growing up, taken by Pappa.

"Pappa, can you take care of my phone?" I ask.

"Yes," He replies.

I hand over my phone and he places it in an inner pocket of his blue lightweight jacket.

My head nurse, Rosa, my anesthesiologist, Dr. Hwang, and Dr. Wazir visit individually.

"Will I wake up during surgery?" I ask the same question to each of them.

"No, that has never happened under my supervision, you will be fine," Rosa, replies.

"You will be fine, you won't feel a thing," Dr. Hwang says.

"Nope, you won't," Dr. Wazir assures me.

"What will be the length of the scar?" Pappa asks Dr. Wazir

"About this much." Dr. Wazir holds up two fingers with a gap of about two and a half inches between them.

Pappa nods and gazes down.

Dr. Wazir smiles and paces back.

Pappa stares at his watch and says it's 7:55 am.

"Alright Mansi, we are ready, follow me to the OR," Rosa says.

I hand Pappa my glasses. Pappa places them in a case and holds it tight in his right hand.

I get up and take a few steps to the doors. I turn back and give Pappa a hug. I inhale his Armani cologne. He rubs my back.

Mummy sprints into the waiting area with her arms wide open and my backpack on her shoulder. Tears stream. She gives me a quick hug.

"Best of luck, Mansi," Mummy says.

I turn around and follow Rosa. I sense Mummy and Pappa's gaze as they watch me go in.

Waking Up

I wake up from my three-hour thyroidectomy. I fell asleep with the thought of escaping.

Bright lights blur my vision. The nurses pick me up and place me onto another bed. I smell disinfectant and hear machines beep.

"You're sweating!" A nurse says.

I look at her and point at my black socks and mumble to remove them. I fall asleep.

"Am I done yet? Do I have a drain on me? What is the time?" I open my eyes again and mumble.

I squint at the clock on the wall in front of me. Pappa has my glasses and phone.

"Yes, you are done. It's 12:30 pm and nope, you don't have a drain," the nurse replies.

I shut my eyes and drift off again.

My throat tightens and feels ticklish. I sit up. The nurse hands me a curved bowl. I hold the bowl with both my hands and hurl into it.

The nurse takes the bowl. I lie back on the bed and fall asleep.

"My neck hurts," I complain with my eyes closed.

"I know," the nurse replies.

I fall back asleep.

"Is it Saegar or Sagar?" I hear a nurse say.

"It's Sagar, it means ocean. She's Indian," says another nurse.

"That's interesting," the first nurse replies.

They mumble, and I try to regain my wits, but I fall back asleep.

I sit up and gag. The nurse hands me a new bowl and my throat forces air out. I hand the bowl back to the nurse.

"My neck hurts," I repeat.

A nurse approaches and checks my vitals. She proceeds to take blood from my inner arm. I feel no pain. I squint and see one cotton-padded adhesive bandage on the back of my right hand, another on my right inner elbow.

I fall back asleep.

Someone nudges me gently.

"Hi, Mansi. I am Joanna, a student surgeon, and I was in the OR during your surgery. I just wanted to inform you…"

I open my eyes and squint at her pink cap. She sits by my bed and smiles. I focus.

"…When we were working on you, your blood went into my eye," Joanna says.

"I'm sorry," I say in my raspy voice.

"It's okay, it's not your fault! Just wanted to ask if we can do an HIV test because of that," Joanna replies.

"Yeah," I reply and fall back asleep.

A few more needles later, I hear heavy footsteps approach.

"Hey, Mansi. How are you feeling?" Dr. Wazir says.

"Tired!" I say, I squint and notice his long beard. "My neck hurts!"

"It's going to hurt. We put you in this position to remove your whole thyroid," he re-enacts the elongated neck position.

"Hmm," I look to my right and my eyes close.

"Take rest," he mutters and walks away.

I wake up with a yellowish fluid pushing through my IV.

"It's anti-nausea medicine, we are going to move you to your ward now," a nurse says.

A few nurses roll my gurney bed. I stare up at the ceiling.

"There's going to be a small bump," a male nurse warns me. The bed shakes getting in and out of the elevator. They pick me up and transfer me to a bed in a recovery ward and the soft pillow touches the bottom of my neck.

"I don't like this pillow. I want my old pillow!" I complain.

The nurses laugh and tuck the old pillow underneath me and adjust the height to help me sleep at an angle.

I squint at the clock in front of me: 2:30 pm.

I fall asleep.

"Why aren't they here?" I glance over at the clock: 2:50 pm.

I hear footsteps approach. It's Mummy and Pappa.

"Where were you? I have been waiting for so long!" I say as I stare at the blurred figures.

They let out faint laughs because they realize I can talk.

"How do you feel?" Pappa asks me as he videos me.

"Sleepy," I reply in my raspy voice.

Mummy places her hand on my head, sniffles, and looks into my tired eyes.

Pappa takes a picture of my neck, his fingers close to my steri-strip. His eyes sparkle with tears as he smiles.

"Your neck is all red," Pappa says.

"What?" I reply.

"I think they cleaned you up with disinfectant, hence the red," Pappa adds.

"Okay," I say.

Pappa hands me my glasses and I put them on. Pappa hands me my phone. I unlock my phone and message Mihir.

"I'm alive," I text. I fell asleep in the OR scared, to the song "Stay" by Alessia Cara and Zedd playing in the background, not knowing if I would wake up.

I video call Kiran Didi and Tanvi Didi. They are surprised to see me talk. I tell them every detail, from the moment I entered the hospital until now. Mummy and Pappa let out faint laughs.

Kiran Didi arrives tomorrow night.

My first nurse walks in.

"Hi Mansi, I'm Kelly, your nurse for the next two hours. Have you had anything yet?" She asks.

I shake my head left to right

"Okay, how about we take a sip of water?" Kelly hands me a Styrofoam cup filled with ice-cold water.

I sip.

Grrrr. I feel my throat makes strange sounds.

"Good job. How does that feel?" Kelly asks.

"It hurts," I reply.

"I know, try eating some Jell-O, we have to get back to normal as soon as possible!" Kelly says.

Mummy opens up the green Jell-O cup and hands me the spoon. I dunk the spoon into the Jell-O and slowly aim for my mouth and swallow. I can feel it scrape my esophagus. My first meal of the day, unless Tylenol Extra Strength counts.

"That's it," I say.

"How about we go to the bathroom and then out for a walk later?" Kelly asks.

I nod.

I sit up and dangle my legs at the end of the bed. Mummy slides on my slippers and I walk to the bathroom a few feet away as Mummy keeps me covered by holding my gown from the back. I waddle with the support of the IV stand. I scan the room; all my neighbors are elderly women.

I get into the bathroom and glance at the mirror. A three-inch white steri-strip covers the incision.

My neck looks smaller.

I am red from my chin to my drooping shoulders. The nurse waits outside. Once I'm done, I waddle out, remove my slippers, and lie onto my bed. I finish my Jell-O, somehow.

I go through my messages.

"You're a lioness, you got this!" One message.

"My lioness, you did it!" Another message.

"Pappa, why does everyone call me a lioness?" I ask him.

"I called you a lioness the first time your siblings came to visit you in the neo-natal ICU. You were fighting for your life." Pappa replies, opens his palms and joins the pinky fingers together. "This is how big you were."

I take a selfie with my neck prominent and post it on my Snap Story with a lion GIF. My hair strands stand out from the perfect bun I tied. My cheeks look puffy. The red makes me look gory.

Kiran Didi jokes I could be Frankenstein for Halloween when I tell her that I have a scar on my neck.

A few moments later Pappa, Mummy and I decide to walk in the hallway. I slide on my slippers. Mummy helps me wear my velvet robe. We let the left sleeve hang empty because of the IV. Mummy ties the robe in the middle, so it stays put.

I hold the IV stand with one hand and Mummy's hand with another.

I ponder how the day started as I waddle from one end of the lit-up corridor to the other.

The Hospital Stay

Look, there they are, Mummy says, as she glances at the end of the hallway.

At 8:00 pm, on the day of the surgery, Pappa, Mummy, and I sit in the visitors' waiting area of the ward, as we wait for Ajay Bhai, my brother, and his family. Metal chairs line the main corridor. Nurses hustle by and elderly patients roam around in wheelchairs.

I spot Ajay Bhai, my sister-in-law Bhabhi, my nephew Aryan, and my niece Avni. Aryan holds a helium balloon which says, "You're So Amazing!" and Avni holds a bouquet of flowers. I smile, they smile back.

"Hi, Mansi," Ajay Bhai says, as he glances at my neck and back into my eyes.

"How are you feeling?" Bhabhi asks. She is two months pregnant.

"Good," I say in my raspy voice.

The kids hand me the bouquet and balloon. I hug them.

Bhabhi takes a seat next to me. Ajay Bhai and the kids stand. They hand falafel wraps to Mummy and Pappa.

"Aunt, what's that?" Avni asks as she points at the IV needle on my hand.

"It's where that goes inside my body." I point to the IV bag.

"What's in there?" Aryan asks.

"Healthy water, filled with vitamins and minerals," I say, as my voice goes up an octave.

Thirty minutes later, I return to my bed and Ajay Bhai and the family leave. I sip the tomato soup they got me.

My third or fourth nurse for the day, marches in, checks my blood pressure and temperature.

At 9:30 pm, Mummy walks me to the bathroom. She helps me brush my teeth and supports me as I waddle back to my bed, then she tucks me in.

"Bye kiddo," Mummy says and kisses my cheek.

Pappa and Mummy head out.

I close my eyes. The nurses approach my neighbor, an old lady—perhaps unconscious. Her beeping monitors distract me. We are separated by a thin curtain.

I sip my water.

I video call Mihir and talk with him 'til I feel drowsy. I hang up the call and doze off amidst intermittent footsteps and beeps.

I feel a sharp pain in my lower abdomen. I check my phone. It's 4:00 am, Tuesday, January 15th.

I shuffle to the washroom, push open the heavy metal door and leave it an inch open. It's difficult to open on my own if it is closed. An elderly lady on the bed opposite the washroom stares at me as I exit. I waddle back to my bed.

I message a heap of friends on Snapchat.

"What happened?" They ask in shock.

"I had thyroid surgery, I had a non-benign lump," I reply.

I want my thick duvet and my murphy bed. I want my view that stretches far out to the horizon from the thirty-seventh floor. I want to count the number of unfocused headlights that pass the intersection nearest to me until my eyes close.

I fall asleep.

At 5:00 am, a nurse tugs at my arm and hands me a small pill.

"Gulp it down, it's your thyroid pill," she says. I think this is my fifth nurse so far.

I look at the pill with one eye closed.

Eltroxin Levothyroxine. The pill my life depends on until I die. I don't have a thyroid gland anymore. Many Google searches and honest conversations will tell you it's no big deal. The butterfly-shaped gland regulates your heart rate, metabolism, energy levels, mood swings and more.

Many people who have thyroid disorders take these and live normal lives. If I don't take this pill regularly, my body will go into chaos-mode, which can lead to various health issues such as fatigue, weight gain, muscle pain, puffy face and more.

I gulp down the pill.

The nurse checks my blood pressure and temperature. I fall asleep.

At 6:30 am a bunch of lab technicians enter with a squeaky cart. A tall nurse adjusts the height of my bed and draws blood from my inner right elbow. She places a cotton ball and adhesive bandage on my arm and moves over to the old lady in the bed next to me.

I press my remote and ask for painkillers. The back of my head and my shoulders throb with pain. I press the button every few minutes.

A nurse arrives with two pills. I force them down.

At 8:00 am, a plump cleaning lady marches in. She beams at me.

"Did you have a thyroidectomy?" She says as she looks at the pile of things on the table next to my bed and back at my neck.

"Yeah," I reply.

"Thyroid cancer?" She asks.

"Got the whole gland removed because it was suspected," I reply.

She sweeps the floor with a broomstick and pan.

"Hmm, it will be okay. You see this scar on my neck?" She says as she points at a faded horizontal scar on her neck.

I nod.

"I had thyroid cancer too...it's no big deal." she says. "I went through radioactive iodine pill therapy later and stayed in isolation and had to shower a lot. It will be over soon."

Radioactive iodine therapy is a targeted therapy to kill off the remaining thyroid cells. It is different to chemotherapy, as the radiation is ingested as a pill, making the person radioactive. This is followed by quarantine for a few days to reduce exposure to others.

"Yeah," I reply.

"Did you know you're not supposed to take dairy an hour after your thyroid pill?" She asks.

"Yeah, my doctor told me," I say as I smile. "What's your name? I'm Mansi."

"I am Victoria...you take rest for now," she says, as she sweeps the floor near the old lady's bed.

Thirty minutes later, I get oatmeal and coffee, my semi-solid breakfast.

I call up Mummy.

"What do you want for lunch?" She asks.

Dr. Wazir walks in.

"Mummy the surgeon is here, I will talk to you later," I say and hang up.

He adjusts the bouquet behind him and takes a seat on the chair. He looks casual in a green t-shirt and running shoes.

"Hey, how are you?" Dr. Wazir asks, as he smiles.

"Good," I reply, as I sip my coffee.

He made me feel safe yesterday in the OR. He patted my face and told me I would be okay.

"How are you holding up with swallowing food?"

"Good."

"Your surgery was successful. We will hopefully discharge you tomorrow. Now, we had to transplant one parathyroid gland, so your calcium levels are low."

He walks over and checks my neck.

"Everything looks good, the white strip should come off on its own. Tell the nurse to remove the knot at the end. I will see you in a month," he says as he smiles, pats my shoulder, and walks away.

I call Mummy again and inform her that my surgeon saw me. I ask Mummy to bring my laptop. I want to get a head start on my reading for class. I message Mihir that my surgery was successful.

I press the remote for my pain killers and they arrive later.

Mummy and Pappa arrive at 10:00 am. Mummy places my laptop on the table beside me.

Mummy walks me to the washroom and gives me a sponge bath. I feel somewhat clean. I want to go home.

Pappa gets me a slice of pizza for lunch and I gulp it down. I feel the hard pizza crust scrape my throat every time I swallow. I ignore it. I want to eat.

They tuck me in and leave.

I stare at my laptop on the table beside me. I don't have the energy to focus on academic language. I turn my phone on. It's 2:00 PM. Nudrat calls.

"Hi, I'm going to be there in thirty minutes," she says and hangs up.

Nudrat has become a close friend over time. We hang out and study together.

She arrives with a basket of chocolates, a "Get Well Soon" card with a butterfly graphic, and a pumpkin scented candle. I beam. She hugs me, and I hug her.

I complain about how IV's aren't fun. I complain about the lady that stares at me. I complain about how it takes forever for my painkillers to arrive.

I press my remote and ask for painkillers. Nudrat goes up to the front desk and talks to a nurse. A nurse arrives soon after with my pills and I gulp them down.

Nudrat helps me put my robe on and we walk outside to the waiting area. We sit on the metal chairs and chat about UTM, hospitals, and about her day.

For a few moments, in Nudrat's company, I forget about the surgery, the IV, and the pain.

Back Home

I'm sorry you have to do this. Thank you for packing up. I'm like a baby. My voice crackles. Kiran Didi flew in from the U.K. with her toddler, Dev, to see me. She helps me put my clothes on and packs my stuff. It's the 16th, the day of my discharge.

A few weeks prior to surgery, My eldest nephew, Jay, who is seven years old, was upset because Dev gets to travel, and he doesn't. He can not travel because he has school. Kiran Didi created characters to help Jay understand. She explained to him that the lump named Bob, the rest of my thyroid named Bobita are bad and need to be removed surgically. Ayush and Aavya, Tanvi Didi's kids, also know about it.

Pappa, Kiran Didi and I wait for my nurse. I want to pull out the IV needle.

My nurse comes in at 11:20 am.

"Okay, let's discharge you. Because of your low serum calcium levels, your surgeon and doctors have advised you to take calcium supplements," she says.

I nod.

"You can take Tramadol, which are narcotic painkillers." The nurse says. "However, try to switch to Tylenol as Tramadol can cause liver problems. Two Tramadol pills every four hours. Also, do you have Eltroxin at home?"

"Yeah," I say, and swallow.

"Okay, do not lift more than two kilograms for a month. You can take a shower but do not apply soap directly to your neck."

"Can you sign this for me?" I ask, as I hand her the form for UTM and she looks it over.

"I don't think I can. I suggest you get it signed by your family doctor," she replies.

She pulls off the adhesive bandage that sits on top of the IV needle on my hand. She removes the needle and applies a Band-Aid.

Kiran Didi helps me wear my jacket, socks, and winter boots. Pappa carries the gift basket Nudrat gave me. Kiran Didi carries the rest of my stuff and I hold her hand. I hold the Styrofoam cup filled with cold water in the other hand. I feel weighed down by my winter clothes.

Passers-by stare as we walk out of the ward.

Kiran Didi and I sit at a table while Pappa waits at the pharmacy to get my prescription. We take a selfie together. I take a picture of her while she holds my "You're So Amazing!" balloon. I send it to Mihir and the WhatsApp family group chat saying that I've been discharged.

"Yay awesome, so proud of you [heart emoji]." Mihir replies.

I send him a heart emoji.

"I am not sure if I want to continue this semester," I tell Kiran Didi.

"Talk to someone about it and then make your decision," Kiran Didi replies.

I call up the Office of the Registrar at UTM and book a

phone appointment for the next morning.

Pappa waves his hand at me and mouths to come over.

"I think Pappa's calling you," she says.

Pappa marches over. I hold his hand and wobble to the pharmacy. I hold Pappa's hand the way I did as a toddler in the bustling markets of Bahrain.

An old lady in a white coat waits for me. She explains what calcium does and how much I need. I zone out. She gets into types of cheeses, yogurts, milk, and butter. I remember only the milk. Three glasses of milk minimum daily.

She scribbles on my prescription while I stare into her stern eyes.

The next day, my eyelids feel heavy, my joints ache, and my neck throbs. I take my pill and wait for the call from Jack, a Financial Aid Officer. My call is scheduled for 9:00 AM. I wait with an empty Word document open.

My phone rings and I jump to answer it.

"Hello, is this Mansi?" Jack questions.

"Yes, I was wondering how will OSAP be impacted if I drop my courses this semester." My voice goes from high pitched to low.

"You will be on probation from OSAP," Jack replies.

"But I just had a major surgery four days ago. I informed the office about this a month before my surgery," I reply.

"If you knew you had to have this surgery, you should have dropped the courses beforehand," he says as he exhales.

"Okay," I mumble.

I agree to whatever he says and end the appointment. I call

up the Office of the Registrar and book another appointment for tomorrow.

Tears overflow, and I wipe them away.

"Mihir, I'm not sure if I want to continue this semester. The guy from the office was not nice," I message him.

"What happened? Do you want me to call you? I'm here," he replies.

"No, don't call me right now," I say and toss the phone on the bed.

I barge out of Mummy and Pappa's bedroom. They prefer I sleep there, as it has an ensuite bathroom. I use my hands on the walls to balance myself as I walk out.

"Pappa, I don't want to do school," I yell at him as tears flow onto my puffy face.

"How can you give up so easily? At least try," Pappa says.

"Mansi, calm down, your stitches will open up," Mummy interrupts as she rubs my back and holds me.

"No," I scream.

Dev, chomping on his breakfast, freezes, and wails.

"Thanks, Mansi," Kiran Didi says sarcastically.

I waddle into the master bedroom. Mummy follows.

"Please don't cry," Mummy says in Gujarati. Tears roll down her cheeks, she sniffles and wipes my face. "Mansi, you just had surgery, stay calm."

"Mummy, I don't want to go to school."

"I know, but we have to be strong. Everyone wants you to be strong, the reason Pappa yelled at you before surgery is because he didn't want to see you weak," Mummy replies.

I weep on Mummy's shoulder. Mummy holds me as she held me when I wept about memorizing multiplication tables in grade two. I lie on the bed and Mummy strokes my hand.

Pappa walks in.

"Where are Mansi's old files?" Pappa asks Mummy.

Mummy searches for the old files and hands it to Pappa. Pappa sits beside me and opens a file.

"You still mad?' Pappa asks.

"Yeah." I wear my glasses.

"Let it go, Mansi...we will figure something out, don't worry," Pappa says.

"Hmm," I reply.

"Look at this," he nudges me and points at a slanted line going upwards, "This was your weight chart when you were at the hospital after birth," Pappa shows me.

I stare at the graph on the old paper.

"Hmm," I say.

"Look at the line going upward, that's your weight. You are a fighter. Don't let school or anything drag you down. We will find a way," Pappa consoles me.

"Okay," I agree with him.

"For now, clear off your mind. Come, let's spend time with Dev outside. School is not important," Pappa says.

I head to the family room and sit there for a while. I return to Mummy and Pappa's room to lie down.

"Try having one pill for now and then we can switch to Tylenol," Pappa insists.

He hands me one Tramadol pill. I agree. One Tramadol pill for the next four hours.

I nod, as I flush the pill down.

Pappa adjusts the pile of pillows that supports my neck. I lean back, message my friends, and scroll through Instagram.

Two hours later, my back hurts. I feel tightness and pain around my incision.

"Hey, how do you feel now? Did you eat?" Mihir messages.

"My neck hurts, you're bugging me," I reply. I lash out at him because my neck hurts. I can feel my stitches throb.

"I'm sorry, I just thought of checking up on you," he replies.

"I want to rest," I reply.

Mihir spams me with inspirational quotes.

"If you need me, I'm here," he says.

I wobble to the family room. Mummy notices and holds me. I sit on the couch. Mummy brings a pillow and I balance the pillow behind my neck and lean back.

"Distract me, I'm in a lot of pain. This is all your fault, the nurse told you two pills. Bad Pappa." I say.

"What movie do you want to watch?" Pappa distracts me.

"I don't know," I say, as I bawl.

"Mansi, you know you can take another Tramadol," Kiran Didi says.

"No!" I yell. "Bad Pappa, this is all your fault! I'm in pain."

"Sorry Mansi, I just want to help," Pappa says.

"The nurse didn't say have just one pill every four hours!" I complain.

"Mansi, you can have another pill, it has been two hours!" Pappa tries to convince me.

"No! I will not listen to you. I want to complete my four hours," I protest.

Mummy and I weep together.

Two hours later, Pappa hands me two Tramadol pills instead of Tylenol and I gulp them down. He feels bad about the situation, so he gives in.

Surprise

Hi, is this Mansi? Sarah, an Academic Advisor, asks, calling me at 9:00 am.

"Yes, hi, just to let you know in advance, I can't talk too loud as I had a thyroidectomy four days back." My voice changes pitches.

"Aww, no worries, how can I help you?" Sarah asks.

"I'm not sure if I want to continue my classes. I spoke to a Financial Aid Officer and he told me the consequences regarding OSAP." I say.

"I suggest you weigh your pros and cons. Take time off, but if you think you are able to continue the semester, then go for it." Sarah replies.

"Okay, thank you," I reply.

Sarah wishes me good luck. I hang up.

I march to the family room without support. I feel better since I switched from Tramadol to Tylenol. I am finally weaned off the opiate pills.

"Hey, how did it go?" Kiran Didi asks.

"It went well," I reply.

"If you want anything, let me know," she says as she sings "Baby Shark" to Dev.

I smile at him and sing "Baby Shark." I wish I could hold him.

I try and WhatsApp call Tanvi Didi.

"Tanvi Didi didn't pick up," I complain to Kiran Didi.

"She probably slept off or is with the kiddos," Kiran Didi says.

"Why are Mummy and Pappa taking so long?" I ask.

"I think they still might be at Pappa's appointment," Kiran Didi reassures me. Pappa said that he has a last-minute appointment this morning.

"Do you want me to get you your glass of milk?" Kiran Didi asks.

"Yes," I mumble.

Kiran Didi gets milk from the fridge and pours a glass. She hands it over. I gulp it down and feel its coolness travel down my throat.

The front door opens and Pappa stomps in. Mummy follows with a smile.

Tanvi Didi barges in with luggage.

"Surprise!" Tanvi Didi yells.

My jaw drops and my eyes water. I hand the glass over to Kiran Didi. I jump out of my sofa and wait for her with open arms. She hugs me, and I hug her. I dig my head into her shoulder and sniffle.

"You came!" I say.

Tanvi Didi flew in all the way from Bahrain to see me.

"It's been six years since we were all under the same roof!" I say, as I look at Kiran Didi and Tanvi Didi.

I call over Kiran Didi and we have a group hug.

"Mansi, you can do this...you are a lioness...go to school in three days," Tanvi Didi says.

"Yeah, university is not a big deal. Since you are already in your courses, try your best. At least you have an excuse if you don't do well," Kiran Didi says.

"I've been saying the same thing!" Pappa adds and lets out a faint laugh.

Tanvi Didi opens her luggage, filled with my favorite childhood snacks and accessories.

I send a picture of chips and baklava to Mihir. I also send him a picture of us three sisters.

"I wish I was there too," Mihir replies.

Mummy and Kiran Didi decide to give me a shower. I take a shower every other day.

Kiran Didi massages and washes my hair. She took care of me as a toddler. She changed my diapers and hid my feeding bottles to annoy me.

Mummy and Kiran Didi switch places. Mummy quickly gives me a shower and helps me dress into my pyjamas. When I was younger, Mummy helped me wash my Rapunzel-like hair.

I walk over to the living room where Tanvi Didi waits with a hairdryer, comb, and hair clips. She's good at hair and makeup. Growing up, I've wanted to be like her.

I sit on the dining table chair. She starts the hairdryer.

Her fingers massage my scalp.

My head and neck ache but I ignore it. I zone out to the loud hum of the old hairdryer.

The next day, we watch DVD's of my fifth birthday party and joke about how I preferred to be fed cake with a spoon. We watch my uncle's wedding video filled with amateur video graphics. Mummy relives her memories of her deceased elder brother and smiles as she watches him dance beside her.

Tanvi Didi, Kiran Didi, and I get identical pastel purple and white bracelets as mementos.

· · ·

One week after my surgery, I attend classes at UTM with a steri-trip across my neck. Pappa drops me off and later picks me up.

Two Point Six Millimeters

So, how are you? Dr. Wazir stands opposite me.

It is early February and I am back at Credit Valley Hospital for my post-op appointment. My legs dangle off the bed. The room is filled with vacant beds and smells like disinfectant. I fidget with my out-patient wristband. Dr. Wazir wears a grey polo shirt with jeans. I glance at his overgrown, salt and pepper beard, then back into his eyes.

"Good...better...tired but I'm back at school." I try to speak up through the intermittent din of the room.

"That's good to hear. So, it was cancer after all," he says, as he exhales, smiles, and purses his lips, "In the five-centimeter lump and in the thyroid, we found two spots. One was two point six millimeters and the other one was smaller. The good news is we got all of it out. We also tested your central lymph node and it came negative."

I swallow hard and glance at my feet. I adjust myself on the examination table.

"We got it out at the right time!" I reply and smile.

"Yeah, you might have to go through radioactive iodine treatment, but your endocrinologist will inform you about that," Dr Wazir says.

"Also, what about this," I say. I play with the thread dangling from one end of my incision.

He scrutinizes my neck.

"Did they not remove this while discharging you?" Dr. Wazir says.

"Nope," I reply.

He gathers a tray of surgical equipment. He puts on gloves, grabs tweezers and pulls out the knot.

"This is what they were supposed to remove," he says as he dangles the tiny knotted thread in front of me.

My eyes widen.

He touches my neck and stares at the sutures.

"Everything looks good."

"One question. What type of cancer is it?" I ask him.

"It's papillary cancer, the most common type of thyroid cancer. Seems like everything's good, your endocrinologist will be in touch with you." Dr. Wazir replies.

"Okay, thank you," I say as I smile.

I gather my jacket and scarf, walk out the doors and gaze at the floor as I approach Mummy and Pappa.

"Let's go," I mumble.

"What did the surgeon say?" Pappa asks.

Mummy and Pappa get up.

"I had or have thyroid cancer…I mean, it's gone, they got it all." I am still in shock.

"What?" Pappa says and freezes.

"The result came back positive for papillary thyroid cancer. One was two point six millimeters and the second one was smaller." I say.

Mummy looks down and Pappa breathes out. We walk with our heads down.

"They did a central lymph node test and it came negative. It did not spread," I say to break the silence.

"What's next?" Pappa asks.

"The endocrinologist will tell me what to do." I reply.

"Hmm…at least it's all gone now," Pappa says as we enter the elevator.

"Yeah, good it's gone," Mummy says.

Moments pass in silence. My eyes water. I look ahead at the empty maze-like hallway.

"The lump was evil!" Pappa says as he lets out a faint laugh. His smile turns into a frown.

I swallow.

"Tell Tanvi, Kiran, and Ajay," Pappa says.

I type a message on the family group chat about what Dr. Wazir said. I forward the message to Nudrat, Mihir, and a few other close friends.

"Wait what? What's next? Let me call you," Kiran Didi replies.

My phone buzzes and I pick up. We enter the elevator at the parking lot.

"Bad Bob. So, now what's next?" Kiran Didi asks.

"I may have to get radioactive iodine treatment done."

"Alright, so the cancer is gone right?" Kiran Didi asks.

"Yeah, all gone," I say as we exit on our parking level and walk towards the car.

"Hmm, keep me posted. I have to cook for Jay and Dev, but I will call you later. Bye," Kiran Didi hangs up.

We reach the car, I jump in, and open WhatsApp.

"Yay, so the bad stuff is out, right? Bad thyroid," Tanvi Didi replies.

"Yeah," I reply. The engine turns on and Pappa reverses.

"So, it's gone right?" Nudrat texts.

"I'm relieved the thyroid was removed at the right time," Mihir replies.

I inform them about the radioactive iodine treatment.

I stare out in the distance as we exit the hospital.

I shiver as I think how I harbored cancer just three weeks ago.

The Butterfly Necklace

On February 14th 2019, I stand by the window in my parents' room. The sun shines on my face. I open Snapchat, choose the fluffy ears filter, extend my arm and take a selfie.

A silver butterfly necklace rests on my neck. Above the necklace lies a still healing, horizontal, two-and-a-half-inch scar.

Two days after my steri-strip comes off, I want to wear a necklace, since I had to take mine off for the surgery. I ask Mummy if I could go through her jewelry. She places the jewelry bag on the bed and takes out gold and silver jewelry. My eyes fixate on the butterfly necklace. Its diamonds sparkle as the sun shines through the window.

"My one-month anniversary of being cancer free," I type and send it to the handful of friends that I trust on Snapchat. I am not ready to open up to everyone just yet, only to my closest people. Snapchat seems ideal, as the stories are temporary, and you can set a timer.

"So proud of you!" Mihir replies.

"Strongest girl out there [heart emoji]." Nudrat replies.

I lock my phone. I remember this day one month back. I swallow hard.

A notification lights up my phone.

My eyes bulge. My throat dries. My eyebrows tense.

"Kareema took a screenshot."

I press on the notification. My eyes well and I clench my jaw.

I message Gina, a close friend I went to high school with.

"Yo, Kareema took a screenshot of my snap...what do I do? I'm upset," I say.

I put my phone away and exhale. Kareema was also a high school friend.

The notification light blinks. I open Snapchat.

"She's so weird. She and I were close friends, but I don't know why she did that," Gina replied.

I pace to my bedroom and hop onto my bed. I sit cross legged.

"Bro, she's gonna send it to people. I didn't want people to find out like this," I reply. I glance at my toes and purse my lips.

"I know, but you shouldn't have sent it to her. Ask her why, if you want to." Gina replies.

I open Kareema's profile.

Why did you take a screenshot?" I message Kareema.

Tears stream. I throw the phone on my bed and it bounces twice before it lands face down.

The golden hour sun blinds my eyes. It's the next day.

"Yo, Kareema still hasn't replied...what do I do? She hasn't even seen my message." I message Gina.

"She takes forever to reply...just forget it. Don't let it get to you," Gina replies.

"How do I not let it get to me? I thought she would respect

it. She took a screenshot instead. I don't want others to find out about my diagnosis like this." I reply.

I go onto Kareema's profile and hit "Block." I pace to the family room and complain to Pappa.

"I have this friend who took a screenshot of a picture I sent on Snapchat to celebrate my one month since surgery," I say as I frown and sniffle. "I don't want to open up like this."

"Mansi, when you send something out to social media, it becomes public. You shouldn't have opened up, if you weren't ready." Pappa says.

I pace to my room and slam the door. I hop onto my bed and look out the large window. The light blue sky turns darker.

I open up Notes on my phone and stare at something I wrote ages ago. I wanted to open up next year. I wanted to create awareness, just not like this.

I turn on my laptop. I open up a blank Word document and type. My nails tap on the keys.

"This picture is of me one-month post-surgery. No makeup. No filters. I don't post personal experiences, and I debated posting this, thinking "What will people say?" but I somehow gathered up the courage and decided to spread awareness.

On January 14th I had a total thyroidectomy (surgery to remove my whole thyroid gland) as I had thyroid cancer. Thankfully it did not spread elsewhere. No cancer is "good" cancer, even if it is treatable. The past four and a half weeks have been physically and mentally exhausting as I lost an important butterfly-shaped gland. It controls good functioning of organs and systems and more.

Wrapping my head around the "C-word" was challenging.

Nobody wants to hear that. It de-railed me and taught me a lot. One thing is the importance of taking care of myself. I planned on posting this in September as part of Thyroid Cancer Awareness Month, but I've changed my mind as awareness shouldn't be reserved for September.

Despite going through a major surgery, I attended class a week later, something that I never imagined I'd be able to do pre-surgery. This was all because of the support I received. I am grateful and thankful for my medical team, family, and close friends who took care of me, supported me, and motivated me by reminding me that I'm a lioness. A fighter. Thyroid cancer got nothing on me!"

My fingers move away from the keyboard. I lean back and exhale. I fidget with the butterfly necklace as my gaze shifts from the computer screen to the horizon. It is night and the fluorescent lights shine. Maybe I should wait.

I copy this paragraph and email it to myself. I copy and paste it on my phone and send it to the Sagar Sisters WhatsApp group. I forward it to Mihir.

I send a picture I took on my one-month cancer-versary of my neck. I wore a baby blue t-shirt and my butterfly necklace. The discoloration from the steri-strip accentuates my two-and-a-half-inch scar.

"Should I post this? Should I open up about my experience? I mean, would you post it?" I send it to Kiran Didi and Tanvi Didi on the group chat. I ask the same to Mihir.

I wait for the responses. I fidget with my butterfly necklace.

"If I were you, I would post this. There's no shame in spreading awareness. There's nothing to hide, you should be proud," Tanvi Didi replies.

"What if people judge me? That I'm a cancer survivor, I don't look like one, I didn't lose my hair. What will people say?" I reply.

"So, what? Let people judge, don't care about their judgments. Post it Mansi, I'm sure Kiran will also agree," Tanvi Didi encourages me.

"Mansi, don't give a damn about what others think. I say do it. Tanvi and I will share it on Facebook," Kiran Didi messages.

"I'm not sure," I reply.

"You can save someone's life," Tanvi Didi replies.

Mihir's notification pops up.

"Absolutely, I'm always here for you no matter what, but this is amazing, and I definitely think you should," Mihir replies.

I pull the blanket over my head and sigh. I am not ready yet.

It's the 17th of February and I dress up for my cousin's daughter's first birthday party. I put on makeup and a red lipstick. I wear my glasses.

My scar stands out. I cannot apply makeup to it.

The butterfly necklace hangs below my scar, the diamonds on its wings sparkle.

I march to the family room and collapse on the couch. Pappa is on his reclining chair.

I unlock my phone and send the paragraph and picture to Pappa.

"Should I post it?" I ask Pappa.

He stares at his phone screen for a minute.

"Yes, post it," he says.

I go onto Instagram, choose the picture, paste the caption and press the "Share to Facebook" icon. The "Post" button comes up. I stare at my screen.

I pace around the family room. My heartbeat fastens. I bite my lips. I grab the butterfly's wing and hold it.

"Do it, what are you waiting for?" Pappa questions.

"Are you sure?" I ask.

"Yes," Pappa replies.

"Are you sure, sure?" I ask again.

"Yes."

"I can't do it. You press the post button," I say, as I pass the phone to Pappa

I press my lips together as I pace in circles. My hands cover my mouth.

"Okay," Pappa says, as he adjusts his glasses, and places his index finger on my phone screen. "I posted it."

He hands over the phone and I message on the Sagar Sister's chat.

"It's done," I say. I forward it to Mihir.

I shut off the screen. I inhale and exhale and wiggle my arms.

An hour later, on our way to the party, Pappa asks Mummy to check the comments as he drives. I stare as cars zoom by on the highway. I hold my butterfly pendant and form a fist.

"You are so...strong," Mummy reads out the comments,

"Thank you for sharing this and bringing awareness. Your experience is inspirational, stay strong. This is real strength...prayers are with you."

I exhale. Goosebumps form and I shiver.

I unlock my phone, read the comments, and exhale. I touch my butterfly pendant, glance down, and smile.

Cancer is Not a Dirty Word

Harpreet and I wait at the bus stop for the St. George Shuttle at UTM on March 15th. It is 4:00 pm. We plan to attend the cancer fundraiser that I asked her to attend together, a month back.

She and I recently started talking again. She reached out to me on Instagram after the surgery post. She was the first friend I made at UTM, but then we got busy with our schedules and lost touch. She is also a thyroid cancer survivor.

I zip up my warm winter jacket and wrap the scarf around my neck. Cold wind blows onto my face as I look at her.

"So how has your health been?" Harpreet asks.

"I've been exhausted all the time, it sucks. Everything aches, and my doctors don't understand that," I reply.

"Yeah, doctors never do. I remember I used to complain a lot after my thyroidectomy," Harpreet nods and glances down. She was diagnosed at the age of sixteen.

I notice a scar from the back of her right ear up to her right collar bone.

"Is that the scar from your surgery?" I ask.

"Yeah, but from my second surgery, I got cancer twice." Harpreet replies, she tucks her hair behind her ear, adjusts her glasses and continues. "It came back. Mine was high risk and I went through two surgeries and two doses of radiation with a gap of a few years."

"Damn, I didn't know," I gulp and look down.

"So, tell me all about it," Harpreet looks into my eyes.

"Long story short, I was really scared to go into surgery. It was a nightmare recovering from the narcotic painkillers. I didn't realize the surgery would change me so much. I get brain fog and I get breathless very easily, especially if I go up a flight of stairs."

"I know it is, but I'm proud of you. You are so much stronger than I was. When is your radioactive iodine therapy?" Harpreet says.

"It's probably during the summer," I reply.

The bus arrives, we enter, and take a seat beside each other.

"I really wish people would understand. You are so brave that you shared your story online, I would be scared," Harpreet says.

"Why?" I ask.

"My parents kept it low, my relatives still don't know. Not even my younger siblings. They were kids when I got cancer," Harpreet replies.

"Hmm, people do react weirdly when you tell them, it's like, taboo," I say.

"Yeah, I know. Apparently, some TA's don't like it either when you tell them about your health issues. One straight up told me to keep it to myself. But I remember Professor McKell told me that cancer is not a dirty word," Harpreet replies.

"I agree with that. Cancer is not a dirty word," I say.

At 6:00 pm, we arrive at the St. George campus and head to the event.

We reach the venue and walk towards the tables swarmed with people wearing blue t-shirts, gossiping and signing others in.

"Hey, we are here for the fundraiser," I approach a girl at the table.

"Hi, are you a volunteer, participant, or a survivor?" She asks.

"Survivors," I answer.

"Cool, I'm Kate, a volunteer. The event is to your right and washrooms to your left straight down," she says as she hands us the yellow t-shirts.

We head for the washrooms. The second I change into the t-shirt, I stand out. Girls entering and exiting stare and smile.

We head to the main event room. As we enter, I notice the blue t-shirts fill up the room. Just two other middle-aged women in yellow t-shirts stand out.

"Dude are we the only young survivors here?" I ask Harpreet.

"Uh-hmm," she replies.

I gulp.

Harpreet and I grab a seat and are approached by volunteers to make paper lanterns. We grab markers, papers, and start working on that.

"Cancer is not a dirty word- Professor M." Harpreet writes on her lantern.

We place the lanterns on the ground in the centre of the room, in a circle.

We grab our seats and continue to talk.

"Alright guys, we are starting our event," a volunteer makes an announcement.

The same volunteer turns on a PowerPoint and starts to thank everyone for participating. The slide shows a picture of a girl. She was also a volunteer. He talks about how she impacted the community and how much she meant to the committee. She passed away recently due to an accident. He wipes away his tears as he speaks.

He moves onto the next slide.

"We are going to start with the survivors walk, can all the survivors come up to the centre, thank you," the volunteer says.

Harpreet and I look at each other in shock. I follow Harpreet to the centre. The lanterns sit in a circle and we form a line around it. The two older survivors stand ahead of Harpreet. I stand behind her.

Marshmello's "Happier" starts and we start our laps around the lanterns.

I follow Harpreet.

My eyes well up and I stare down at the different lanterns. I scrutinize the words and colours. Tears flow down my cheeks as I follow Harpreet and I sniffle.

I hold my hands over my mouth.

"Are you okay? I didn't even notice you were crying," Harpreet whispers, as she glances back.

I turn back, and the blue shirts join behind me. I wipe away my tears and take deep breaths.

We scatter back to our spots.

"I'm alright, I just didn't think I would cry. I felt overwhelmed." I say.

"I was not expecting this. I hate it. All I wanted to do was fundraise, not feel framed as a survivor. This is a pity party," Harpreet adds.

I nod.

Harpreet and I grab our free pizza slices and munch.

"If I ever get hired for them, this is the first thing I'm changing," Harpreet complains, as she eats her pizza.

I nod as I gulp.

"We aren't survivors like these t-shirts say. Warriors would have been a better word," Harpreet says.

We finish the pizza slices, change back to our normal tops, and head back to the UTM bus stand.

Acknowledgements

In early 2019, while I was recovering from my thyroid cancer surgery, I contacted Sujaya Devi, a former WRI420 student and the author of "Write Left" on how I could create my own book. I wanted to share my story.

In May, I discussed my idea with Professor Guy Allen. I wrote out my content over the summer with Professor Robert Price and Professor John Currie.

I would like to specially thank Professor Allen for his guidance and trust.

I would like to thank Nick West for polishing my writing 'til it turned out right.

I would also like to thank Celine Polidario for designing a beautiful cover.

Without Nick and Celine's hard work and dedication, this book would not be how it is today.

I would like to thank all my friends, acquaintances, fellow WRI420 classmates, professors, and family members who have motivated me to keep going. Your support has meant a lot.

Lastly, I would like to thank Pappa and Mummy for being my backbone. Thank you for believing in me and teaching me that whatever I want to do can be possible, if I put my heart, passion, and efforts into it.

About the Author

Mansi Sagar is an Indo-Canadian writer, a thyroid cancer "warrior", and will be graduating from the University of Toronto Mississauga in November 2020. She was born and brought up in Bahrain, lived in the U.K. during her early teens, and immigrated to Canada in her mid teens.

Mansi struggled with communicating in English growing up. She got into fiction writing in school in the U.K., where she realized she enjoyed writing pages and pages of stories for English class. This led to her pursuing writing as a major.

In university, Mansi created a self-help blog called "Rediscover Yourself" to share her experiences of growing up with depression, anxiety and not fitting in. The blog can be accessed at https://sagarnexgen.wordpress.com/ .

Mansi hopes to use her writing to break taboos and spread awareness.